AROMATHERAPY & ESSENTIAL OILS

FOR

BEGINNERS

Discover the Phenomenal Powers of Essential Oils to Relax, Revitalize, and Revolutionize Your Health

(Create Your Holistic Wellness Spa at Home Book 1)

<u>NEW, REVISED EDITION</u>

By Marta Tuchowska

Disclaimer:

If you are suffering from any serious or chronic disease(s) or condition(s), or if you are on medication (even if natural, e.g. homeopathy), please consult with a medical or naturopathy doctor (or other health professional, if applicable) before you start using aromatherapy. Natural therapies are very safe to use, but please keep in mind the precautions that are included in this book. Not all the aromatherapy treatments are safe for women who are pregnant, so please consult with your doctor/midwife/ and/or aromatherapist first. Always check the safety information supplied with any new oil, research the brand, and make sure that the products you buy for your home spa are 100% natural and organic.

Contents

Introduction

I want to thank you for taking an interest in the book: *Aromatherapy and Essential Oils for Beginners (Holistic Wellness Spa at Home Part 1)*. It really means a lot to me! I am excited to be sharing my holistic spa secrets with you and help you increase your quality of life with natural wellness treatments.

This book is a practical guide on how to create your own personalized holistic spa. You will discover the pleasure that comes from creating various aromatherapy natural treatments for your body, mind and spirit. You will learn about all of the benefits that the therapeutic essential oils and other herbs can offer. Aromatherapy is not only about the beauty treatments; it can also alleviate various common ailments related to stress.

I would like to add that this book is not only for women. Real holistic spa is about restoring balance- something that everyone is seeking for in their very own way. So, for my male readers, do not deprive yourself of creating your spa at home. You may even learn some really handy skills so as to impress her with your knowledge of aromatherapy and holistic facial massage.

You will be amazed to discover that essential oils can have multiple health benefits. Moreover, you will realize that the natural solutions described in this book will be very affordable, eco-friendly, and easy to use. After a hard day at work you really deserve a nice, relaxing evening at home.

Discover the healing and energizing properties of aromatherapy, wellness and holistic beauty treatments that this book describes. Creating your home SPA can also be a great idea for a rainy weekend when you stay in or want to socialize with your family and friends. Why don't you try something new and *really* healthy?

You will also develop fantastic skills that you can then practice on your family and friends. The peace, balance, energy, relaxation and wonderful aromas of your home SPA will bring about the ultimate holistic wellness experience for you and your loved ones. I have selected my favorite aromatherapy oils, as well as other ingredients, that will give you the chance to create a range of treatments

for various conditions and imbalances, such as skin and hair conditions, water retention, digestive problems, cellulite, colds,
 as well as anxiety, stress, insomnia, frustration and anger. Even if you do not suffer from any of the above-mentioned conditions you can still benefit from this book and take even better care of your health and beauty.

Now...Let the holistic spa journey begin...
So, take a few deep breathes, put on some nice relaxing music and maybe spice it up with some incense sticks and...have a nice read! Have a break whenever you need to and don't forget to practice what you have learnt. Let's DIVE INTO IT.

Chapter 1 Your Holistic Wellness SPA

Are you looking for an affordable way to relax at home? Create your very own holistic wellness SPA! Everybody loves getting treated at luxurious spas, but some spa treatments can be very expensive. All you need to get started on your holistic wellness home spa is a couple of essential oils, vegetable carrier oil, or a natural cream. As for the other ingredients, you probably have most of them in your kitchen. You can access highly personalized treatments with the healing aromas very inexpensively. Are you ready to create your home spa? Fortunately, you won't have to create your own products. Instead, you will simply mix various aromatherapy oils to relax your body and soothe your mind. But first things first:

What is a holistic spa ?

The word *holistic* comes from the Latin word *holisium*, which means *entire, all, whole.* The objective of holistic therapies is to restore balance where there is imbalance with the aid of natural therapies alone. All holistic practices and therapies encourage a person to take control of their health and their lifestyle by looking inside themselves and correcting certain unhealthy habits. For example, instead of just taking a pill to mask a problem, the holistic approach tries to get to the root of the problem. What causes pain, stress, and anxiety? Why is it so difficult to relax?

The questions for you are: Are you willing to take responsibility for your health? Are you willing to invest your time in learning how to relax so that you can improve your health holistically and feel better physically and mentally?
Taking on some new healthy habits will bring magnificent health benefits in the long run! Relaxation skills are the best defense against disease!

What is wellness?

Wellness is the sensation of feeling stress-free, having optimal energy levels, and being free from disease. There is a healthy balance of the body, mind and spirit that results in happiness and a feeling of connectedness with the "here and now".

Creating your home spa will definitely help you to experience the holistic wellness sensation and feel rejuvenated. Moreover, you can *create* it whenever you want and wherever you want. All you need to do is to put your mind to it.

What are the benefits of creating your home spa?

More men and women are looking for products that have not been tested on animals. You might want to ask yourself the questions below to determine whether a home spa is for you:

-Are you fed up with false claims of beauty marketing methods?

-Are you concerned about pollution?

-Are you interested in self-reliance and living a simple life? Do you like to 'do-it-yourself'?

-Do you love natural herbs, spices, and oils and enjoy their fragrances?

-Do you enjoy learning new, creative skills?

-Are you horrified at the amount of synthetics in commercial skincare and beauty products?

-Are you interested in natural therapies for relaxation?

-Would you like to learn how to fight headaches, migraines, insomnia and some common complaints naturally?

If you answered *yes* to at least 5 of those questions, it means that you are very motivated when it comes to looking for new eco-friendly solutions and taking care of your health holistically.

Drawbacks of using chemical beauty products

-They have no benefits for the mind.

-They can contribute to many illnesses.

-During the process of their production the chemicals leach into the soil and contaminate farmland.

-Some of these products may cause allergic reactions or other skin problems.

If you think that stress-management is something that only therapists should know, you are wrong. Everyone should be continuously learning new techniques to fight/reduce stress. It has been scientifically proven, that if unmanaged and uncontrolled, stress can lead to a diminished quality of life, as well as:

-Anger, sorrow and many other negative emotions

-Inability to control personal and professional life

-Anxiety and insomnia

-Digestive problems

-Depression

-No zest for life and no focus

-Decreased immunity

Do you really want to succumb to stress, or do you prefer to maximize your wellbeing instead?

The natural treatments complete with the relaxing fragrance of aromas will definitely help you cope with stress. You will fell in love with your very own holistic spa, and creating it at your home will become an inseparable ritual in your life. If you are a therapist or are familiar with some spa treatments, then I hope that this book will help you get inspired to relax more. From my experience, I know that all spa professions normally involve long hours of really hard work in order to help others improve their well-being and eliminate pain. Massage therapy also requires lots of dedication, concentration and physical work.

This is why, in my opinion, all therapists should also take some time to take care of themselves, relax and 'pamper themselves' whenever they can, so as to always be at their best and do high quality work treatments on their clients.

This book may also encourage you to become a holistic therapist or do a certified training in natural/holistic/massage therapies. If you are already in love with wellness, you will soon realize that one passion will lead you to the next, in other words: there is no end to this amazing world of natural therapies and massage.

I hope that this book will give you enough inspiration to create something unique to you, your needs and your expectations. Listen to your intuition and your creativity and let them guide you.

Chapter 2 What is Aromatherapy?

After discovering aromatherapy and all the benefits of it, I completely stopped using the commercial chemical beauty products and I switched to natural aromatherapy oils and organic creams. I was fascinated by the fact that I could use essential oils for a whole range of treatments. For example, geranium oil works for oily skin, edema, water retention, and cellulite. It also has many mental health benefits: it fights migraines, reduces anger and anxiety, and even provides better sleep.

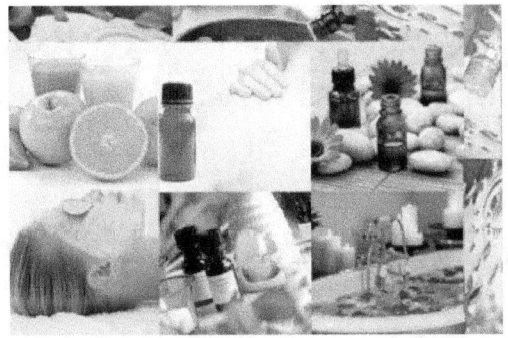

As you will see, aromatherapy is a truly holistic therapy and a single treatment can have multiple benefits for your body and mind.

Aromatherapy- what exactly is it?

Aromatherapy can be defined as a holistic treatment that brings a physical, spiritual, emotional and mental sense of wellbeing through:

-Inhalation of aromatherapy oils
-Massage with aromatherapy oils
-Aromatherapy bath.

Aromatherapy formed part of healing and beauty rituals of many ancient cultures. In fact, it was a sacred practice in ancient Greece, Egypt and Rome, as well as in India and China. It was also practiced by Mayans and many other ancient civilizations.

Julius Cesar was given a daily aromatherapy treatment to help alleviate his neuralgia condition. Many diseased or injured people were treated with aromatherapy massage, as ancient Indian, Chinese and Greek manuscripts recount.

How does aromatherapy work?

This wonderful stress-relieving therapy can be used in different ways:

1. By entering the circulatory system via the skin through massage (especially recommended for sore muscles, skin or hair conditions)

The oils are absorbed into the bloodstream (this is why it is so important that they are natural) and once in the circulatory system their properties (e.g. balsamic, anti-fungal or anti-bacterial) start working and healing.

2. Through the lining of the lungs through inhalation or vaporization.

The soothing scent of oils affects the limbic system in the brain via the olfactory tract. It has a wonderful effect on nervous and hormonal systems. It also reduces negative emotions and improves memory and concentration.

Aromatherapy has been scientifically proven to produce wellbeing and harmony as well as to improve health and prevent many stress-related conditions.

A Mini Disclaimer on other ways of using Aromatherapy:

Internal use of essential oils is another way of employing aromatherapy. This branch of Aromatherapy is often called Phytoaromatherapy and many sources refer to it as *Scientific Aromatherapy*. Phytoaromatherapy treatments are not normally practiced in spas and so they won't be included in this book. However, its therapeutic power cannot be overlooked and I would like to offer some general views of it:

The pure essences diluted with olive oil, or cane sugar and taken internally are very effective treatments for respiratory problems, digestive problems as well as anxiety and insomnia.

Phytoaromatherapy is very similar to Herbalism and if you are looking for specific treatments for your condition or illness, then only after a detailed consultation will the Aromatherapist can they be able to design a treatment for you. Aromatherapy, Herbalism or other Natural Therapies should never be equaled to self-medicating. The fact that they are natural does not mean there are no precautions; an experienced therapist will be able to advise you of the perfect treatment in perfect synergy, doses and duration.

In the case of taking essential oils internally, it is extremely important to make sure that the oils are labeled organic and contain their chemo-type on a label.

Very important- not all essential oils can be ingested. Then, not all brands qualify as pure and organic enough to use this form of application. Most brands offer essential oils that should not be ingested. However, if you are interested in learning more about this form of application, I recommend you google: Pranarom. It is a really good, organic brand from Belgium. They have lots of useful info on their website and offer trainings and books. Disclaimer- I am not affiliated with this company.

If you are interested in aromatherapy it is also worth mentioning here the different schools of aromatherapy:
-The French School of Aromatherapy
-The British School of Aromatherapy

Different countries follow different schools of aromatherapy, whereas some countries adapt more of a mixed approach, (this is what I do personally). They tend to compete a lot as they stress different approaches when it comes to employing aromatherapy treatments: **The British School of Aromatherapy excludes** the oral intake of essential oils and stresses the importance of aromatherapy massage (essential oils diluted in carrier oils in 2, 5-5% concentrations). It mainly focuses on balancing emotions and mood but also uses aromatherapy to alleviate certain conditions of a more physical nature.

The French School (The above mentioned brand-Pranarom represents the French School), on the other hand, **includes** the oral intake of essential oils and defines itself as a scientific branch of aromatherapy. It also includes using aromatherapy topically, but very often in concentrations that are higher than 5%(essential oils diluted in a base vegetable oil).

I originally got my diploma in Aromatherapy with The School of Natural Health Science,(International College of Holistic Medicine). That is the British School approach, and after moving to Spain, I discovered that there was much more for me to learn, as many local schools and courses promoted *Scientific Aromatherapy* and I trained in that as well.

Now, I like to I combine the knowledge that I gained from both the British as well as the French School of Aromatherapy and personally I believe that both approaches are highly therapeutic. The reason why I mentioned the differences between the two schools is that very often, according to resources that you use, you may come across a different approach.

For example, as mentioned before, some therapists exclude taking the essential oils internally (as if it was completely verboten, but in reality, it's all about learning about the safe mode of application- never experiment with ingesting EO if you are not too sure how to go about it-safety first). My intention is to make you aware that different approaches do exist so as to avoid any possible confusion when you come across something that wasn't mentioned in this book.

Aromatherapy is a really broad topic. There are certainly many ways of employing it.

If you are an advanced aromatherapist and would like to know about the internal use of essential oils, I recommend that you learn more about Scientific Aromatherapy from the following resources:

-*Chymotyped Essential Oils* by A.Zhiri, D.Baudoux, M.L. Breda

You can google it to find it in your local online store. I think it's available in different languages.

The Spa World tends to adapt more of a British School approach, which is more simplified, and this is what I also follow in this book. After all, it's a beginners' guide.

What is the difference between essential oils and vegetable oils?

Contrary to their name, essential oils are not oily at all. They are pure essences obtained from petals, flowering tops, leaves, roots and wood of various plants and trees. Essential oils can never be applied or massaged in their pure form because they may cause allergic reactions. The only exception is if you use a drop of your chosen essential oil on your wrists as if it were a perfume and then inhale the fragrance, as you might do for headaches, general relaxation at the workplace or when you travel(it is always more advisable to dilute them with a few drops of a vegetable oil though).

Vegetable oils serve as a base for essential oils to be diluted. This is why they are very often called base oils or carrier oils. Vegetable oils are also used for massage. The most popular are sweet almond oil, avocado oil, sesame oil, and hazelnut oil. (You can read more about vegetable oils in Chapter 4.)

How should I mix essential and vegetable oils?

The general rule that I recommend is:
For 15 ml of your chosen vegetable oil use 5- 8 drops of your favorite essential oil(s).

To make things easier, 15 ml equals 1 tablespoon.

When dealing with physical problems, e.g. sore muscles, you can make the mixture stronger and add a few more drops of your chosen essential oil (e.g. rosemary, clove and basil essences are great for sore muscles or for athletes).

However, when dealing with problems more emotional in nature, e.g. anxiety, depression, and insomnia, it is recommended to use no more than 6 drops of essential oils per 15 ml vegetable oil.

For example, if someone is suffering from anxiety and tension headaches, I recommend a gentle neck massage with the following mixture:
1 tablespoon of a vegetable oil+ up to 4 or 5 drops of lavender, or: basil/ mint/ verbena/ or bergamot.

You can also mix different oils together. For example: 1 tablespoon of a vegetable oil+ 2 drops of lavender+ 2 drops of bergamot + 1 drop of other essential oil(so it's 5 drops in TOTAL)

or: 1 tablespoon of a vegetable oil+ 1 drop of lavender+ 1 drop of basil+ 1 drop of verbena+ 1 drop of mint+ 1 drop of bergamot.(so it's 5 drops in TOTAL)

You will find out more about recipes and essential oils' properties in the following chapters.

Can I mix the essential oils with other creams, lotions or face masks?

Yes, of course you can! If the products that you are using are organic, you can do the following:

1. Add one drop of your chosen essential oil to your face cream or facemask.

For example, geranium is great for oily complexions, but it is also known as sebum-regulating oil, so it can be also used for mixed or even dry skins. Ylang ylang is a great skin tonic especially for mature skins whereas palmarosa is great for dry skin and tea tree oil is recommended for acne. Moreover, all of these oils work as natural remedies for headaches and mental exhaustion. If you have sensitive skin, try the mask on your wrists first to make sure that there is no allergic reaction.

2. Add one or two drops of your chosen essential oil to your shampoo. Rosemary, juniper, and grapefruit are great for preventing hair loss and also stimulate hair growth.

My tip:
In the summer I prefer to use natural aloe vera gel rather than vegetable oils. The reason for this is that aloe vera is absorbed quickly into the skin and has a nice cooling effect. Mixed with the energizing mint essential oil, it has a strong refreshing effect, something truly recommended for hot summers.

I suggest you make sure that the products you use as a base are natural and organic.

Aromatherapy Precautions

-In case of serious conditions or if you are on medication please consult with your doctor or a local aromatherapist first before using aromatherapy;

- If you are undergoing a homeopathy treatment, abstain from using mint and chamomile essential oils;

- If you are undergoing any natural treatment (e.g. floral, herbs, Chinese, etc.) consult with a naturopathic doctor or a herbalist first before using aromatherapy;

- If you are pregnant. Do not use aromatherapy without consulting it with your local aromatherapist. Some essential oils are safe during pregnancy, but it is always recommended that you consult with your therapist or a doctor first;

-Do not use on infants (unless you consult it with your local aromatherapist or a doctor that is specialized in natural treatments as well);

-For children use blends in lower concentration and preferably consult with your local aromatherapist or naturopathic doctor first to obtain a personalized treatment advice;

-Do not use the blends on damaged skin;

-Avoid contact with the eyes;

-All essential oils should be kept away from heat and direct sunlight. Keeping them in the fridge will make them 'live' longer;

-Avoid sunbathing after applying the oils (especially in case of citrus oils: bergamot, lime, orange, grapefruit, etc.);

-Remember that the essential oils once diluted with carrier oil will only last a few weeks. I recommend preparing your mixtures in small amounts just for specific treatments. If, for practical reasons, you wish to make and store your blends, I recommend that you keep them in mini glass bottles and store them in the fridge.

-Do not apply undiluted.

The results of aromatherapy are almost immediate...It is also very easy to get started on. If you want to bring more joy, pleasure and happiness into your life, just confide in aromatic oils and let them work for You and your wellness!

Chapter 3 Essential Oils for Beauty and Health

Now you know what aromatherapy is. You have learned how to differentiate essential oils from vegetable oils. You also know how to mix the oils.

Congratulations! You have just finished the most difficult part, and you can now get started on the more pleasurable aromatic and practical part.

Simply read this chapter and chose your favorite 3 essential oils. Then get them at your local aromatherapy store or order them online. Make sure that the oils you buy are of good quality and organic. There are lots of companies producing synthetic mineral oils rather inexpensively, but these oils have more drawbacks than benefits and we don't want them at your home spa.

They may have some nice aromas, but they don't have any therapeutic properties that we are looking for. This is why I suggest you always double-check and select only certified, organic oils. You should be very careful about what you put on your skin. Essential oils are considered to be very effective because they also work from the inside. Of course, they must be natural, not just some cheap synthetic oils.

In this chapter, I have listed some of my favorite essential oils.

There are actually hundreds of them. Aromatherapy is a life-long study, but the essential oils I mention will quickly open the door to the whole range of treatments. They also offer various fragrances and properties that can be adapted for your highly personalized beauty and relaxation treatments.

Here are a few additional very important precautions to keep in mind:

- After an aromatherapy massage- always remember to wash your hands;

- Make sure that you research the brand, read safety instructions for each individual oil you buy/use and check the expiration date;

- Store your blends in dark glass bottles, preferably in a cool, dry and dark place and remember to use within a maximum of one month after mixing;
- Do not apply oils after surgery (unless you have consulted with a doctor) or on open wounds or rashes of unknown origin;

- Do not use the oils after chemotherapy (unless suggested by a doctor);

- Keep the oils away from the eyes and mucus membranes;

- Use the oils only topically (unless you have consulted with an aromatherapist who specializes in phytoaromatherapy);

- Avoid rosemary, thyme, Spanish and common sage, fennel and hyssop if you suffer from high blood pressure;

- Do not apply the treatments described in this book on babies or infants. It doesn't mean that aromatherapy can never be used on babies and infants, but extremely low concentrations should be used. Always consult with a medical or naturopathy doctor first.

Bergamot (*Citrus Bergamia*)

It has a great, fresh, fruity, orange-like smell. It was actually named after the Italian city of Bergamo, where it was first discovered and sold.

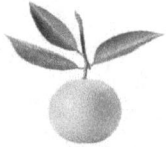

Therapeutic Indications:

For the Body

-Skin care: acne, boils, cold sores, eczema, insect repellent and insect bites, oily complexion, psoriasis, scabies, spots, varicose veins

-Respiratory system: sore throat, tonsillitis

-Digestive system: flatulence, loss of appetite (apply a gentle abdominal massage)

-Immune system: colds, fever, flu

For the Mind

-Anxiety, depression, anger, insomnia

-Stress-related conditions, lack of energy to cope with problems

Safety/Precautions

-phototoxic when exposed to direct sun light

Cedarwood Atlas (*Cedrus Atlantica*)

It has a sweet, woody-balsamic fragrance and is also well-known as an aphrodisiac.

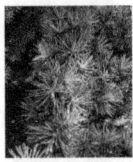

Therapeutic Indications:

For the Body

-Skin care: acne, dandruff, dermatitis, eczema, fungal infections, oily skin, hair loss, skin eruptions

-Circulation, muscles and joints: arthritis, rheumatism

-Respiratory system: bronchitis, catarrh

For the Mind

-It is an amazingly soothing tonic for the nervous system, and it's recommended for stress-related conditions and nervous tension. It brings inspiration to artists and writers.

Safety/Precautions

-non-toxic, non-irritant and non-sensitizing but better to be avoided during pregnancy (unless consulted with your doctor or health provider)

German Chamomille (*Matricaria Recutica*)

The plant has an apple-like relaxing scent that eliminates stress and anxiety.

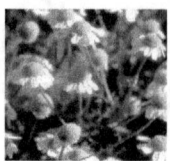

Therapeutic Indications:

For the Body

-Skin care: acne, allergies, boils burns, cuts, chilblains, dermatitis, eczema, hair care, inflammations, insect bites, and rashes

-Circulation, muscles and joints: arthritis, inflamed joints, muscular pain, neuralgia, sprains, rheumatism

-Digestive system: nausea, indigestion (via gentle abdominal massage)

For the Mind

-Headache, insomnia, anger, nervous tension, migraine, and stress-related complaints

Safety/Precautions

-It may cause dermatitis in some individuals, but overall safe, non-toxic and non-irritant

Cinnamon (*Cinnamomum zeylanicum*)

It has a sweet, spicy scent and is considered to be a very powerful aphrodisiac. It can also be mixed with clove or ylang ylang essential oils that are well known for their aphrodisiac properties.

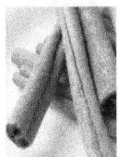

Therapeutic Indications:

For the Body

-Skin care: Lice, warts, wasp stings

-Circulation, muscles, joints: poor circulation, rheumatism

-Digestive system: anorexia, colitis, sluggish digestion

-Female wellbeing: childbirth (stimulates contractions), frigidity

-Immune system: chills, colds, flu

For the Mind

-Debility, emotional breakdown, nervous exhaustion, lack of focus

Safety/Precautions

-may cause irritation to mucous membranes, be sure to use in moderation

Citronella (*Cymbopogon Nardus*)

It has a powerful and uplifting lemony scent. I like to use it as a natural energy booster and whenever I feel tired or exhausted, citronella oil can really 'sort it out' and restore my balance.

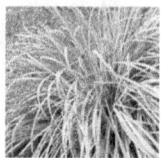

Therapeutic Indications:

For the Body
-Skin care: excessive perspiration, oily skin, insect repellent
-Immune system: colds, flu, minor infections

For the Mind
-Nervous system: Fatigue, headaches, migraine, neuralgia, feeling overwhelmed and tired, lack of motivation

Safety/Precautions
-it may cause dermatitis in some individuals
-avoid during pregnancy
-avoid sunbathing (phototoxic)
-non-toxic/ non-irritant

Cypress (*Cupressus Sempervirens*)

It has a sweet-balsamic tenacious odor.

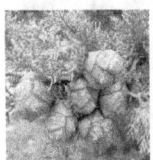

Therapeutic Indications:

For the Body

-Skin care: oily and over hydrated skin, excessive perspiration, insect repellent, varicose veins

- Circulation, muscles and joints: cellulite and edema, muscular cramps

-Respiratory system: spasmodic coughing

-Female well-being: menstrual pains (apply with a gentle abdominal and lower back massage)

For the Mind

- Disperses negative emotions, helps to make positive changes, helps in treating nervous tension and fighting stress

Safety/Precautions

-non-toxic, non-irritant and non-sensitizing but perform a patch test if you have a really sensitive skin

Frankincense (*Boswellia Carteri*)

This scent is used by many spiritual gurus for meditation purposes and it helps focus the mind and achieve the inner balance.

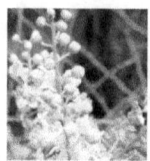

Therapeutic Indications:

For the Body

-Skin care: blemishes, dry and mature complexions, scars, wounds, wrinkles

-Respiratory system: asthma, bronchitis, catarrh, coughs

-Female wellbeing: menstrual pain

For the Mind

-A great remedy for anxiety, nervous tension and other stress-related conditions. It helps the mind achieve a deep meditative state and combats negativity.

Safety/Precautions

-good news: non-toxic, non-irritant, non-sensitizing

Geranium (*Pelargonium graveolens*)

It has a rosy-sweet, slightly minty scent that is relaxing and uplifting.

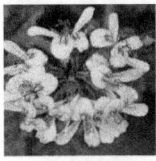

Therapeutic Indications:

For the Body

-Skin care: acne, bruises, broken capillaries, burns, congested skin, oily complexion, mosquito repellent

-Circulation, muscle and joints: cellulite, water retention, muscular tension

-Respiratory system: sore throat

For the Mind

-Relieves feeling of overwhelm, stimulates ideas, reduces stress and mental exhaustion; recommended for students

Safety/Precautions

-it may cause dermatitis in hypersensitive individuals

-otherwise non-toxic, non-irritant + non-sensitizing

Grapefruit (*Citrus x paradise*)

It has a wonderful, energizing scent that will lift even the laziest spirit offering a well-deserved body and mind detox!

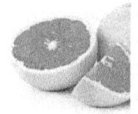

Therapeutic Indications:

For the Body

-Skin care: acne, congested skin, hair loss, thin or damaged hair, oily scalp

-Circulation, muscles and joints: cellulite, muscle fatigue, obesity, stiffness, water retention. Used by sportsmen as a preparation for exercise

-Immune system: chills, colds and flu

For the Mind

-Mental exhaustion, depression, headaches

Safety/Precautions

-non-toxic, non-irritant, non-sensitizing

-better to avoid direct sun exposure after applying

Ylang ylang (*Cananga odorata var. genuina*)

It has a strong floral smell that some people love and others can't stand! Personally, I don't like strong floral scents, but I recognise the remedial benefits of ylang ylang. It is a great aphrodisiac, but first make sure that your partner can tolerate flowery scents. If not, I suggest that you choose cinnamon or clove instead.

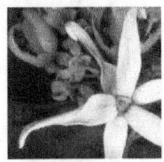

Therapeutic Indications:

For the Body
-Skincare: acne, hair growth, hair rinse, irritated skin,
-Circulation, muscles and joints: high blood pressure, abnormally fast breathing, palpitations

For the Mind
-Fights frustration and helps to overcome past traumas and experiences, limits negative emotions, increases intuition, reduces feelings of anger, sorrow and internal confusion. It is recommended for writers and artists to get some inspiration.

Safety/Precautions
-non-toxic and non-irritant if used in moderation
-may irritate the mucous membranes

-may cause headaches or even nausea if overdosed

Allspice (*Pimenta dioica*)

As its name suggests, it has a strong, sweet-spicy scent. It was traditionally used as a natural pain killer and muscle relaxant. This oil will make your home spa a 'health' spa, especially in the winter, as it has strong anti-flu properties.

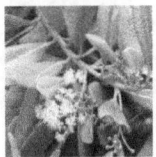

Therapeutic Indications:

For the Body

-It is a great natural remedy for circulation, muscles and joints: it helps alleviate muscle cramp, stiffness and arthritis pain

- A gentle chest massage with oils containing a few drops of allspice oil helps alleviate cough and fight flu

-Digestive system: indigestion and flatulence

For the Mind

-It's helpful in cases of mental fatigue

-Recommended for cases of neuralgia, depression, tension and stress

Safety/Precautions

-may irritate the mucous membranes

-better used in low dilutions only

Angelica *(Angelica archangelica)*

The Angelica plant with all its kinds and varieties is widely employed by the Chinese as it is well known for the whole range of healing properties like e.g stimulating the immune system, revitalising the spirit and promoting fertility. It has a spicy, herbaceous scent that stimulates the body and mind.

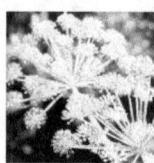

Therapeutic Indications:

For the Body

-Digestive System: lack of appetite, flatulence, indigestion

-Skin problems: irritated skin, psoriasis

-Immune system: colds, coughs, sinusitis

-Circulation: water retention, accumulation of toxins

-Muscles and joints: rheumatism

For the Mind

-Stress-related conditions, nervous breakdowns, tension headaches

Safety/Precautions

-not safe for diabetics and pregnant women

-the root oil may be phototoxic

It is time to get pampered!

Find your local aromatherapy provider and order the oils that you think your body and mind need.

Experience the sensation of aromas. How does it feel? Which oils do you prefer? To which oils do you naturally get attracted? Use your intuition! Put a drop or 2 of a pure essential oil on your wrists whenever you feel that stress is at the door. Does it help? Can you actually smell and feel the therapeutic properties of the aromas? How about adding a few drops to your bath or enriching your cream or body lotion? The next step is to read Chapter 4 and learn more about vegetable massage oils. You can use them in your blends for all the creative and intuitive stress-releasing self-massages!

Chapter 4 Vegetable Carrier Oils

Vegetable carrier oils are famous for their hydrating properties and form part of many natural beauty treatments. They also work as a base for diluting essential oils. As you already know, the pure essence can't be applied without any vegetable oils. Let me just give you a few examples of my favorite vegetable oils, I want you to remember though that there are hundreds of them and so I always encourage you to explore them as much as you can:

1. Sweet almond oil:

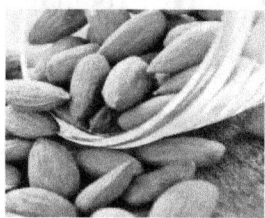

This oil is very kind to the skin and light in texture. The oil is extracted from the seeds (nuts); oil from the bitter almond is not used. It is extremely rich in fatty acids and is therefore great for moisturizing preparations, as body milks, reconstructing night creams, hand creams or softening treatments (e.g. feet).

2. Argan oil: This oil is native to Morocco and became very famous in the last couple of years and many beauty professionals (hair dressers, beauticians, etc.) recommend it for regular hair or skin care. It is quite expensive but if you use it in its pure, natural form you won't have to use big quantities of it. It contains a lot of alpha tocopherol (a form of vitamin E) and has very strong skin-softening properties. It can even reconstruct damaged hair or skin and reduce wrinkles. I use argan oil as a night cream substitute, especially in the winter. It also works miracles for my hair giving it a healthy shine (you will find more instructions at the end of this chapter).

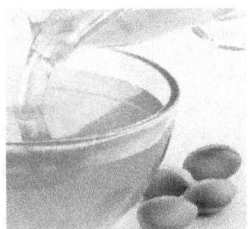

3. Avocado oil: Avocado oil comes from Central America. It is now known world-wide and is very popular as massage oil. It has a light green color and is good for rehydrating skin, elasticity, and skin regeneration. Dry, fragile and sensitive skin will benefit from avocado oil. Some people may be allergic to almond or sesame oil, so avocado oil is a much safer option.

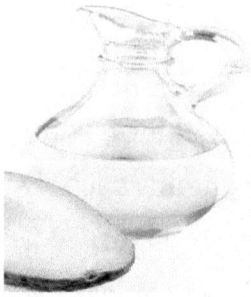

4. Jojoba oil: This oil is extracted from the seed. The best kind is gold color and cold pressed. It can be used in anti-ageing treatments as a hand cream, body cream, hair conditioner or after sun lotion. It's excellent for chapped skin.

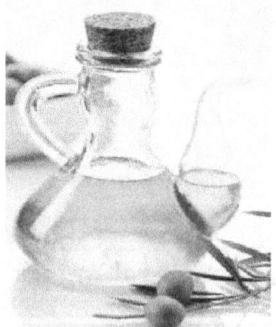

*As you can see, the jojoba oil can be confused with olive oil. Jojoba plant's fruits also look a bit like olives...

5. Hazelnut oil: This oil is extracted from the nut and has a nice nutty aroma. It is rich in vitamins A, B, and E and is famous for its softening properties. It is recommended for hair treatments (especially dry hair). It has reconstructing properties and is great for skin, nails, hair, etc. It is also widely used as an ingredient in sun lotion products.

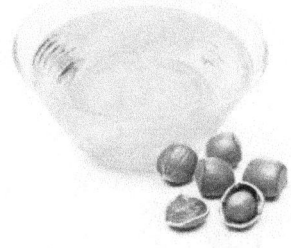

Exercise: Order at least one vegetable carrier oil so that you can start mixing it with your essential oils. Remember the golden rule: one tablespoon of a vegetable oil needs about 5- 8 drops of an essential oil. Try to mix various vegetable oils and simply experiment with them! You can also use the vegetable oils without mixing them with any essential oils. Vegetable oils are a great alternative to skin moisturizers, creams and lotions, and hair conditioners.

*A note on jojoba oil: many resources refer to it as *a wax,* as technically it is a wax, however nowadays many therapists call it *jojoba oil* and you can also find this term in many resources. *No matter how you decide to call it though,* you can still use it!

How do I use vegetable oils to recover damaged hair or to prevent hair loss?

All the vegetable oils that I mentioned are great for hair loss prevention as well as for hair recovery (bleached or dyed hair). However, there are some oils that are especially recommended if you want to re-grow your hair and make it lustrous. Try castor oil, coconut oil or babassu oil (great for dry, brittle and damaged hair).

It's simple: you just mix the vegetable and the essential oils of your choice in a little glass bowl and apply the mixture on your head via gentle scalp massage. Also apply on the hair. Avoid head massages on wet hair. It is better to apply the mixture on dry hair before you wash it. Massage your scalp using quick movements that apply pressure. Leave in for at least an hour. For best results leave it in overnight and wash it in the morning using a gentle herbal shampoo. For oily scalps I suggest that you apply less oil and instead of working mainly on the scalp, focus more on the hair. However, if you use some essential oils like geranium, lemon, bergamot (also effective for dandruff treatments), you will regulate sebum secretion.

If done regularly (once or twice a week) natural oil treatments will speed up hair growth and improve hair density. Apart from a natural and effective hair treatment, you will also relax holistically as scalp massage eliminates tension accumulated due to stress or emotional overload.

It is time to create your Beauty Spa with highly hydrating vegetable oils...You can invite some of your favorite essential oils to make your treatments even more pleasurable!

Chapter 5 Body & Mind Recipes

Try some of my body and mind recipes at your home spa!

They will de-stress and rejuvenate your body, mind and spirit in a truly holistic manner.

Holistic Wellness Spa Blends

For relaxation:

-15 ml base oil + 2 drops of ylang ylang + 2 drops of bergamot + 2 drops of sandalwood

To apply:

-Gentle neck and shoulders massage or full-body massage is recommended.

-Aromatherapy bath

To fight muscular aches and pains:

-15 ml base oil + 2 drops of marjoram + 2 drops of rosemary + 2 drops of ginger

To apply:

-Use the blend to massage the areas affected.

To fight headaches:

-15 ml base oil + 1 drop of lavender + 1 drop of peppermint + one drop of marjoram

To apply:

-Gentle facial massage as well as neck massage is recommended.

To fight anxiety, anger and stress:

-15 ml base oil + 2 drops of lavender + 2 drops of geranium + 1 drop of sandalwood

To apply:

-Gentle face or head massage, including neck and shoulders, is recommended.

-Aromatherapy bath

To fight cellulite and water retention:

-30 ml base oil + 2 drops of cypress + 2 drops of juniper + 2 drops of lavender + 2 drops of rosemary + 2 drops of orange + 2 drops of lemon + 2 drops of fennel

To apply:

-Massage the legs, starting with the ankles and moving up. You want to make sure that you follow the direction of the venous circulation.

For athletes:

-40 ml base oil + 3 drops of clove + 3 drops of lavender + 3 drops of rosemary + 3 drops of ylang-ylang

To apply:

-Legs, arms and back massage
-Aromatherapy bath

To fight insomnia:

-15 ml of base oil + 2 drops of lavender + 2 drops of chamomile + 1 drop of mandarin

To apply:

-Face massage, neck massage or full-body massage
-Aromatherapy bath

For dry skin:

-15 ml of base oil + 2 drops of sandalwood + 2 drops of palmarosa + 2 drops of rose

To apply:

-Gentle facial massage. It is a great night cream alternative!

For mature skin and wrinkles:

-15 ml of base oil + 2 drops of frankincense + 1 drop of myrrh + 2 drops of palmarosa

To apply:

-Facial massage, apply before going to bed.

For acne:

-15 ml of base oil + 2 drops of geranium + 1 drop of cedar wood + 2 drops of bergamot

To apply:

-Facial massage, apply before going to bed, use this treatments at least 3 times a week

For hair loss prevention and to stimulate hair growth:

-15 ml base oil + 2 drops of juniper + 2 drops of ylang ylang + 2 drops of grapefruit

To apply:

-Head massage, leave in for at least an hour and then wash your hair with a gentle organic shampoo

Try Cleopatra's style aromatic bath:

How to prepare an aromatherapy bath and optimize its therapeutic effects:

Add 5- 8 drops of your aromatherapy oils (in total) to a glass of milk. Add to your bath only when the water is not running. Breathe in and relax!

Combine Aromatherapy with Hydrotherapy and bring balance where there is imbalance...

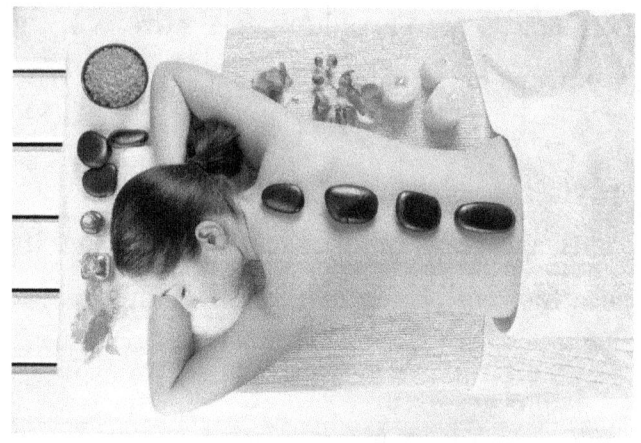

* Hippocrates, the father of medicine, strongly advocated the use of therapeutic plants and herbs as well as their healing essences. According to his teachings, to enjoy a

strong and healthy life one should bathe in aromatic waters regularly and treat oneself to a daily massage with scented oils...

I would add that if Hippocrates was to see the fast-paced 21st century world, he would probably recommend multiple aromatic baths/treatments a day, not just one!

Let's face the truth...who isn't addicted to their phone, social media accounts, plus...the list of modern electronic gadgets goes on and on...

Luckily, almost an immediate relief is always there for us as long as we are willing to take action to actually relax!

In this day and age, Hippocrates' teachings are as needed as never before...Let's put theory into practice...

Hopefully while finishing this chapter you are already preparing your aromatic bath to revitalize holistically!

Chapter 6 Facials, Herbs and Other Natural Treatments

Apart from aromatherapy oils I also recommend that you try some rejuvenating herbs and other natural ingredients. You will be able to create affordable and eco-friendly solutions for you home spa. You probably have most of these ingredients in your kitchen already. Creating your own products means that you can tailor your product to your skin type and other personal characteristics and preferences. Your imagination and knowledge is the limit of what you can do.

Avocado:

Mash and mix with 1 teaspoon of honey, a squeeze of lemon juice, and a drop of your essential oil to personalize according to your skin type. This can be used for headaches.

Banana:

Mash and mix with 1 teaspoon honey plus a few drops of sweet almond oil or olive oil and enrich with some essential oils if you wish. (Use no more than 2 drops per mask.)

Infusions for oily skins:

Use 1 or 2 teabag size per cup, cool down and use as a skin tonic, apply only fresh: yarrow, parsley, mint, fennel, sage, blackberry leaves

Infusions for dry skin:

Use 1 or 2 teabags per cup, prepare an infusion, cool it down and use as a skin tonic. Apply only when fresh. Chamomile, honeysuckle, angelica and rose infusion are great natural tonics for dry skin.

Natural Yoghurt:

Smooth on and leave in for 15 minutes. Rinse off with tepid water. It is great as an after sun treatment! You can add one drop of the essential mint oil to cool the skin down. You can also use it to fight tension headaches.

Oats:

Mix with some hot water, cool down in a fridge, and add some vegetable base oil (e.g. jojoba, olive oil or sweet almond oil). To personalize, spice it up by adding up to 2 drops of your favorite essential oil.

Here are some recipes, but designing your own is the fun part...

Honey and lavender moisturizing mask:

It is also great to reduce stress, fight anxiety, and ward off insomnia.

1 tablespoon of organic honey + 2 drops of lavender essential oil + 1 tablespoon of Argan Moroccan oil

Strawberry and Rosemary rejuvenating face mask:

It is also great for sinusitis, low energy levels, anger and headaches.

1 drop of rosemary essential oil + 1 drop of chamomile essential oil + a few mashed strawberries+ 1 spoon of green clay (or honey)

Green clay mask for oily skin:
It is also great for headaches, insomnia and depression.

2 tablespoons of green clay + 1 drop of bergamot essential oil + 1 drop of verbena essential oil + 1 tablespoon of honey

Enjoy, and remember not to limit yourself with the experiments. If you have sensitive skin and are prone to allergies, test the mask first by applying it on your hands or wrists. Wait half an hour to see if there is an allergic reaction.

Going red? For sensitive skin (like mine, which goes red after the majority of face mask treatments, even natural ones) use yoghurt, aloe vera gel, chamomile essential oil (only 1 drop) and prepare natural skin tonics. Mint, chamomile and rosemary infusions are great for that. Apricot kennel vegetable oil as well as jojoba oil can also be used for sensitive skin. Aloe vera soothing gel is one of my favorites, regular guests at my home spa beauty rituals. Not only is it great for my sensitive skin but it also regulates sebum secretion and so it is a great 2 in 1 treatment for skins that are oily and sensitive. Try it yourself!

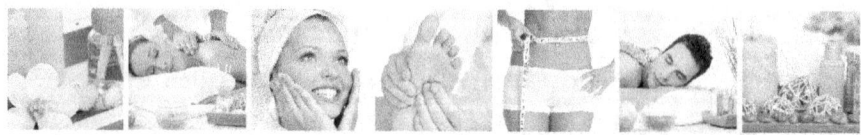

Chapter 7 Setting the Scene

In order for you or the recipient of your treatment to relax, you need to make sure that you set a nice, relaxing scene for your spa. All the details are important:

-Make sure that there is no noise and switch off your mobile phone and other devices. You don't want to get distracted. It is your time and your treatment. You need to disconnect, and so does your mobile phone!

-If you don't live on your own, let your family or your roommates know what you are planning to do. Ask them not to disturb you. It is your personal relaxation time. Alternatively, you can also ask them to join you. Preparing aromatherapy blends and exchanging simple intuitive massages can be a great therapeutic experience. It is also a great alternative to just sitting around and watching TV...

-Playing some gentle music will create a sense of tranquility and calmness. It is better to avoid energetic beats.

-Select a fragrance that you like. Select your aromatherapy essential oil and add a few drops to an oil vaporizer with a little water. Geranium and lavender are my favorites as they stimulate the feeling of relaxation. You can also use Indian Ayurvedic incense sticks.

-Soften the lights or use candles. Prepare the towels before the treatment and have everything at hand. You can also play with the colors of the towels. Color therapy is also included in many luxurious spas.

-Prepare the pillows, hair bands, cotton wool pads and cucumber slices if you wish.

-Perform a few deep diaphragmatic breaths and stretch! Breathe consciously but don't force it, just let it come! Breathe in imagining the energy filling your body and breathe out getting rid of all the stress, pain and negative emotions.

If there are any negative thoughts or day's events coming to mind, don't worry about them. Just accept them and repeat to yourself:

It is time for me to relax. No people and no events can spoil this moment! I am taking responsibility to take care for my body and mind. Tomorrow I am going to wake up full of energy and I will be able to solve all my problems. I am good at solving problems because I know how to relax!

Stretch intuitively and direct your conscious breathing to all the pain and tension affected areas. Stretching is a form of self- massage and you will also stimulate your lymphatic system, which is responsible for increasing your immunity levels and eliminating toxins and bacteria.

Just by paying attention to breathing you can access new levels of health and relaxation that will benefit every area of your life. - Deepak Chopra. An Ayurvedic doctor, philosopher and healer.

Chapter 8 Juices and Teas to Rejuvenate

What is the secret of the most luxurious spas in the world?

It is simple: not only do they pamper their clients with aromatherapy massages, but they also offer organic teas and juices to help them detoxify. It is not only about massage and treatments from the outside. It is also important how you feed your body from the inside.

While aromatherapy treatments or natural masks are doing their jobs or while you are taking your aromatherapy bath, you may be interested in trying out some of the following caffeine-free teas and juices. Remember that some herbal infusions as well as fruits can also be used in natural beauty treatments.

I have already mentioned that some infusions, such as rosemary and mint, act as skin and hair tonics. But they also offer more benefits. The majority of the people just drink their coffee or black tea and forget about the herbal kingdom of therapeutic infusions. Also keep in mind that caffeine abuse adds to anxiety, tension, insomnia and exhaustion.

Try some if the following infusions at your home spa. For your increased health and relaxation, try:

1. Oatstraw infusion: to reduce fear and anxiety.

2. Mint and chamomile infusion: to de-stress and to sleep better.

3. Rosemary infusion: to prevent colds and flu and to increase your energy levels.

4. Banana+ blueberries +spinach +coconut milk smoothie: for better circulation, more energy, detoxifying treatment as well as to have healthy skin and hair.

5. Carrot+ spinach+ grapefruit juice: for a healthy 'slightly tanned' skin. It is also a natural anti-ageing treatment.

6. Pineapple + blueberry + coconut water + green tea smoothie: for better digestion, to fat burn and to reduce cellulite.

7. Mint + apple + blueberries + kale +vegan milk (coconut, almond) smoothie:
for better circulation, as well as to fight edema, cellulite and water retention.

8. Valerian infusion: to relax the nervous system, fight anxiety and ward off insomnia.

9. Horsetail infusion: to promote strong hair and to reduce water retention. It is also recommended in weight loss diets.

10. Carrot+ cucumber + lemon juice: to eliminate toxins and to stimulate the lymphatic system.

11. Red tea or green tea: to burn fat and get more antioxidants.

12. Banana+ coconut milk+ coconut oil + chia seeds smoothie: to strengthen the nerves and get more energy.

It is time to create your very own Home Health Spa with highly revitalizing natural home-made juices and herbal infusion. Restore your energy naturally and avoid caffeine drinks, you will be amazed at the results!

Chapter 9 Bonus Chapter: Holistic Facial Massage & Mindfulness

This bonus chapter will take you on a marvelous holistic journey of facial massage with essential oils. Now, that you know how to mix the oils I strongly recommend you take advantage of what facial massages can offer! You will also learn some basic techniques to get started on body and mind rejuvenating relaxation.

Mindfulness will be the word to describe the greatly holistic state of wellness you will find yourself in in less than a few minutes...

Simple steps to perform a holistic facial massage(on yourself or on others):

The techniques suggested come from Swedish Massage, Neurosedative Massage and Indian Face Massage.

1. Mix the oils and apply small amounts at a time. Gently stroke the face with the pads of your fingertips. Do it slowly but try to maintain a steady rhythm. This gentle stroke is called neurosedative touch and it stimulates relaxation. Breathe in deeply, hold it for a few seconds, and then breathe out slowly.

2. If needed, apply some more oils to make sure that the skin is moist enough to do a massage, but avoid over applying oils as your hands would then be losing contact with the skin. If the area gets too slippery, it's harder to do the treatment.

3. Using the area of the hand just below the thumb (the mound at the base) try moving your hand in circles around on the forehead. This technique will eliminate accumulated tension. Work on the forehead and then move to the temples, cheeks and chin area. The jaws can also accumulate great amounts of tension. If you feel any knots or tension, work the affected area a bit longer. Follow your intuition also as it tends to be much more effective than following massage protocols (which are good for getting started). Repeat a few times, doing one side at a time: work on the left, then the right side of the face. Keep switching.

You may notice that one side of the face has more accumulated tension than the other. This is normal.

4.Using your fingers of both hands, gently make circles on the skin around the forehead, then move to the temples area and down to the jaw and chin area.

5. Using the pads of your fingers, gently squeeze the eyebrows and keep increasing the pressure. This technique is best performed employing your middle fingers and the thumbs. It also brings a great relief to a frontalis muscle and prevents migraines and headaches.

6. Using all your fingers - the pads of your thumbs plus the pads of the rest of the fingers - gently squeeze the chin and then move up to the jaws area. You may also want to experiment with moving your jaw to release tension.

7. Pressure points - For this technique, you will be using the pads of your thumbs (or middle/index fingers, whichever works best for you) pressing different points on your face to enhance the therapeutic and healing effect of the massage.

Ayurvedic Massage and Shiatsu and Chinese Acupressure are all disciplines that work with these powerful points to stimulate healing. I only present an extremely simplified review of some of the oriental manual therapies, but you will be amazed at the results.

Each point should be worked on for about 10-15 seconds and then released, and the whole procedure can be repeated again on the same point. Focus on the points that bring an immediate relief to you or your recipient as well as points that accumulate pain or tension. (This is a sign of some inner imbalance that can be healed with manual therapy.)

- Apply gentle but firm pressure to the middle of the forehead between the eyebrows. This point is called the Third Eye in Ayurvedic Medicine. *Then* work the eyebrows, simply applying the pressure on the points following the eyebrows line and stopping on the point where the eyebrows finish. Press it using the same technique and then work the temple areas. Applying pressure there can bring relief if you suffer from sinusitis.

- From the temples, start moving up following the hairline. According to Chinese acupressure, working on the hairline is an inseparable part of a face or head massage as it brings focus, concentration and calms nerves at the same time.

When your two hands meet in the center of the hairline, you can also apply the pressure to your scalp following the middle line. Get back to the hairline using the same path and move down to the *third eye* again and apply pressure.
- After working the *third eye*, apply pressure under the eyes in line with the pupils and hold for 10- 15 seconds. From there, move your hands down and work the corners of the mouth. There are pressure points approximately 1 inch away from the corners of the mouth.

- Gently rub the earlobes.

Going through the steps described above will bring feelings of relaxation and focus. Moreover, you can always skip the oils part and simply do the pressure points part, which is a great solution if you are at work or have limited time. If you do it on someone else, they will almost certainly ask you to do it again!

You can also practice the following technique to stimulate holistic relaxation:

- Hold your hands out in front of you. Your palms should be facing each other but not touching at all. Allow your hands to close very slowly. Concentrate on your breath. Breathe in deeply and breathe out slowly. Choose your own rhythm and bring all your attention to your hands, let them move away and bring them back close, but make sure that they are not touching each other. After several repetitions you may start experiencing the sensation of warmth between your hands and this sensation may be spreading on to your body. This is what many therapists and reiki practitioners call *healing energy*. If you don't feel anything, don't worry about it but focus on your breathing and imagine a big ball of energy, like the Sun, between your hands.

- Slowly move the ball of energy up and place it on your head. Put your hands on your head, relax, keep breathing and imagine the cascading energies of light that enter your body through your head and spread into all directions. You may want to concentrate on the areas that are in pain, or even on certain emotions that need healing.

- Finally stroke your face, arms, legs and the whole body, and to finish, shake your hands off, imagining the dust that is leaving your body so that the healing can occur. Simply keep practicing when needed, listen to your body and your intuition. For optimal results, try the techniques described in the chapter at least twice a week. Facial massage can be performed anywhere, you can even do it in your office. The use of oils can be optional, and you can just simply focus on working on the pressure points.

Conclusion

Thank you again for downloading and reading my little *SPA* book! I hope you enjoyed aromatherapy and other powerful, natural body and mind treatments that I have covered. I also hope that I managed to inspire you to take a well-deserved spa break. A holistic spa break that you can create anytime, wherever you want and really inexpensively.

The next step is to use your imagination and create your holistic wellness spa at home. Try your own spa rituals and relax when you need it. Spread relaxation and rejuvenation for your loved ones the way they deserve. Make Holistic Wellness Spa something more than just beauty or relaxation treatments- make it *your lifestyle*!

Until next time we "meet", wishing you all the best on your wellness journey,

Much love,

Marta

About Marta

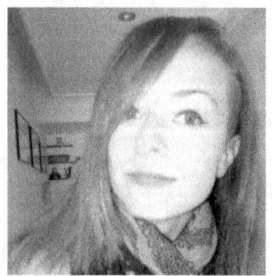

Marta Tuchowska is a passionate holistic wellness author on a mission. She wants to help you create a healthy body, mind and spirit through a balanced lifestyle. Marta has a strong background in healing and health (certified in massage therapy, holistic nutrition, aromatherapy and Reiki), and she infuses her natural therapy knowledge with motivational and life coaching to help you create a life full of energy, health and happiness. Marta wants to make it easy, doable and fun. She calls it holistic lifestyle design for modern, 21st-century, busy folks! Join the exciting journey of total body and mind transformation at: www.HolisticWellnessProject.com.